RECOGNIZING

RELATIONSHIP

RED FLAGS

A Guide To A Healthy Love

MELISSA J. POWELL

TABLE OF CONTENT

6. Emotional Well-being

6.1 Emotional Manipulation

6.2 Gaslighting

6.3 Constant Criticism or Belittling

7. Financial Compatibility

7.1 Financial Secrets or Irresponsible Behavior

7.2 Incompatible Financial Goals

8. Intimacy and Affection

8.1 Lack of Intimacy or Affection

8.2 Withholding Affection as a Punishment

8.3 Incompatibility in Sexual Preferences or Frequency

INTRODUCTION

Recognizing red flags in a relationship is crucial for maintaining emotional well-being and fostering healthy connections with others. Whether you're in a new relationship or a long-term one, identifying warning signs early on can help you make informed decisions about your future. In this guide, we'll explore the common indicators of unhealthy dynamics and provide insights on how to navigate them, ultimately empowering you to build more fulfilling and harmonious relationships.

CHAPTER 1

Introduction

1.1 Why Recognizing Red Flags Is Important

1.2 The Impact of Ignoring Red Flags

1.1 Why Recognizing Red Flags Is Important

In the complex tapestry of human relationships, recognizing red flags serves as a critical compass guiding us towards healthier and more fulfilling connections. Whether we're in the honeymoon phase of a new romance or deeply entrenched in a long-term partnership, understanding and identifying these early warning signs can be the difference between thriving and suffering in our relationships.

Red flags are subtle, yet significant signals that something may be amiss in a relationship. They are the cautionary whispers of doubt that often go unnoticed or are dismissed in the initial stages of emotional involvement. However, learning to recognize and address them is paramount, as doing so empowers us to make informed choices about our future.

At the heart of why recognizing red flags is important lies the pursuit of emotional well-being. Healthy relationships should uplift and support us, providing a safe space for growth, trust, and love to flourish. When we ignore red flags, we risk jeopardizing our emotional health and happiness.

1.2 The Impact of Ignoring Red Flags

The consequences of overlooking these early indicators of trouble can be profound, affecting both our mental and physical well-being. Let's delve into the various aspects of life where the impact of ignoring red flags becomes evident.

1.2.1 Emotional Toll

Ignoring red flags often leads to emotional turmoil. As we suppress our concerns and doubts, we become entangled in a web of denial and self-doubt. This emotional distress can erode our self-esteem and self-worth, leaving us feeling trapped and helpless.

Unaddressed red flags can also fester, creating a toxic environment where resentment, anxiety, and sadness thrive. In such situations, emotional intimacy and trust deteriorate, robbing us of the joy and connection that should be the bedrock of any healthy relationship.

1.2.2 Erosion of Trust

Trust is the cornerstone of any meaningful relationship, be it romantic, familial, or platonic. When red flags are ignored, trust becomes compromised. As doubts and suspicions linger, they can poison the trust that once bound partners together.

Over time, a lack of trust erodes the foundation of the relationship, making it difficult to communicate openly and honestly. This breakdown in trust can manifest in secrecy, jealousy, and constant doubts, leading to emotional distancing and, ultimately, the deterioration of the relationship.

1.2.3 Physical and Mental Health

The impact of ignoring red flags extends beyond emotional distress, taking a toll on our physical and mental health. Prolonged exposure to a toxic relationship can lead to stress-related health issues such as insomnia, depression, and anxiety disorders.

In some cases, individuals may resort to unhealthy coping mechanisms, such as substance abuse, as a way to numb the pain and frustration stemming from unresolved red flags. This not only jeopardizes their well-being but also deepens the chasm in the relationship, creating a vicious cycle of dysfunction.

1.2.4 Stifled Personal Growth

Healthy relationships should foster personal growth and self-discovery. However, when red flags are ignored, personal development often takes a backseat. The energy and effort spent on managing relationship issues detract from self-improvement and can lead to stagnation.

Moreover, individuals in such relationships may find themselves isolated from their support networks, as red flags often result in the alienation of friends and family who witness the unhealthy dynamics. This isolation further stifles personal growth and prevents individuals from seeking the help and support they need.

In Conclusion

Recognizing and heeding red flags in relationships is a vital skill for anyone navigating the intricate terrain of human connections. Understanding the importance of these early warning signs is the first step towards fostering healthier and more fulfilling relationships.

By ignoring red flags, we inadvertently invite emotional distress, erosion of trust, and harm to our physical and mental health. Moreover, we risk stifling our personal growth and potential.

In the sections that follow, we will delve deeper into the common red flags that may surface in various types of relationships and provide guidance on how to address them constructively.

Empowered with this knowledge, we can embark on a journey to create and sustain relationships that are characterized by love, respect, and mutual well-being.

CHAPTER 2

Communication

2.1 Lack of Open and Honest Communication

2.2 Frequent Misunderstandings and Miscommunications

2.3 Unwillingness to Discuss Future Plans

Certainly, let's delve into the topic of communication, specifically addressing three critical aspects: the lack of open and honest communication, frequent misunderstandings and miscommunications, and the unwillingness to discuss future plans. Effective communication is the bedrock of healthy relationships, both personal and professional. It serves as the glue that binds individuals together, facilitates understanding, and fosters collaboration. When communication falters in any of these aspects, it can lead to a cascade of problems and complications.

2.1 Lack of Open and Honest Communication

Open and honest communication is the cornerstone of any successful relationship. Whether it's between spouses, colleagues, friends, or family members, the ability to express thoughts, feelings, and concerns openly is paramount. Unfortunately, a lack of such communication can breed mistrust and resentment.

In many cases, individuals may withhold their true thoughts or feelings due to fear of confrontation, rejection, or judgment. They may resort to passive-aggressive behavior or simply choose silence over confrontation. This lack of transparency can create a wedge between people, preventing them from resolving issues and understanding each other's needs and desires.

In the workplace, a lack of open and honest communication can manifest in various ways. Employees might hesitate to provide feedback to their supervisors, fearing repercussions or creating tension. This reluctance stifles innovation, productivity, and growth within the organization. Similarly, managers who fail to communicate openly with their teams may leave employees feeling undervalued and disconnected from the company's mission.

2.2 Frequent Misunderstandings and Miscommunications

Misunderstandings and miscommunications are almost inevitable when open and honest communication is lacking. These issues arise when information is unclear, incomplete, or misconstrued, leading to confusion and frustration.

In personal relationships, misunderstandings can occur over trivial matters or escalate into significant conflicts. For example, a simple miscommunication about plans for the weekend might lead to disappointment and resentment if not addressed promptly. Over time, repeated misunderstandings can erode trust and intimacy.

In a professional setting, miscommunications can have serious consequences. A missed email or an unclear directive can lead to costly mistakes, missed deadlines, or damaged client relationships. The repercussions of these errors can be far-reaching, impacting an organization's reputation and bottom line.

2.3 Unwillingness to Discuss Future Plans

The third aspect we'll explore is the unwillingness to discuss future plans. This issue can be particularly detrimental to long-term relationships and organizational success. When individuals or groups avoid discussing their future goals and aspirations, they often find themselves heading in different directions, which can lead to dissatisfaction and conflict.

In personal relationships, couples may drift apart when they fail to have open conversations about their individual and shared dreams. One partner may be envisioning settling down and starting a family while the other is focused on career advancement and travel. Without honest discussions about these desires, resentment can build as each person feels their needs are being ignored.

Similarly, organizations can suffer when leaders and employees are not aligned in their visions for the future. A lack of communication about long-term goals and strategies can lead to confusion and disengagement among team members. Employees may struggle to see how their individual contributions fit into the larger picture, resulting in reduced motivation and productivity.

In conclusion, communication is the lifeblood of relationships and organizations. The lack of open and honest communication can give rise to numerous problems, including misunderstandings, miscommunications, and an unwillingness to discuss future plans. Addressing these issues requires a commitment to transparent and empathetic communication, a willingness to listen actively, and a genuine desire to understand and meet the needs of others. By fostering a culture of open communication, both personal and professional relationships can thrive, and organizations can achieve their goals with greater success.

CHAPTER 3

Trust and Honesty

3.1 Consistent Dishonesty or Omissions

3.2 Trust-Breaking Behavior

3.3 Privacy Invasion

Trust and honesty are two fundamental pillars of any healthy relationship, whether it be between individuals, within families, or in the context of professional associations. These virtues serve as the bedrock upon which strong bonds are built. In this discussion, we'll delve into the various facets of trust and honesty, with a particular focus on consistent dishonesty or omissions, trust-breaking behavior, and privacy invasion.

3.1 Consistent Dishonesty or Omissions

Consistency is key in any aspect of life, and this holds true for trust and honesty as well. Consistent dishonesty or omissions can be highly detrimental to a relationship. When one party repeatedly fails to provide truthful information or withholds important details, it erodes the foundation of trust that the relationship is built upon.

Trust is, essentially, a belief in the reliability, truth, or ability of someone or something. When consistency in honesty is lacking, that belief is shattered. It becomes difficult to rely on or have confidence in the person who consistently engages in dishonest behavior.

Moreover, consistent dishonesty can have a domino effect, leading to a spiral of mistrust and suspicion. Once trust is broken in one aspect, it tends to affect trust in various other areas as well. For instance, in a romantic relationship, if one partner repeatedly lies about their whereabouts or finances, it can lead the other partner to question their commitment, intentions, and even the overall validity of the relationship.

To rebuild trust in the face of consistent dishonesty, open and honest communication is crucial. Acknowledging one's past mistakes and demonstrating a genuine commitment to change are important steps in the right direction. However, it's important to remember that rebuilding trust takes time, and there are no shortcuts. Trust, once broken, cannot be fully restored overnight.

3.2 Trust-Breaking Behavior

Trust-breaking behavior encompasses a wide range of actions or choices that directly undermine the trust someone has placed in another. These behaviors can vary in severity, from minor breaches to actions that cause profound damage to a relationship.

Examples of trust-breaking behavior include infidelity in a romantic relationship, betrayal of confidences, stealing or deception in financial matters, and failing to meet commitments or promises. In each case, these actions can lead to a breakdown of trust, often with far-reaching consequences.

In romantic relationships, infidelity is perhaps one of the most severe trust-breaking behaviors. It not only involves dishonesty but also a breach of commitment and loyalty. Recovering from such a betrayal can be incredibly challenging and may require extensive efforts on the part of both parties involved.

In the realm of friendships, betraying confidences by sharing personal information or secrets without consent can be equally devastating. Trust is built on the understanding that what is shared in confidence remains confidential. Once that trust is violated, it can be difficult to regain.

The road to rebuilding trust after trust-breaking behavior is a difficult one, and it often requires deep reflection, remorse, and a willingness to make amends. In some cases, professional counseling or therapy may be necessary to facilitate the healing process.

3.3 Privacy Invasion

Privacy is a fundamental human right, and respecting someone's privacy is closely intertwined with trust and honesty. Privacy invasion occurs when one person intrudes into another's personal space, accesses their private information without consent, or crosses boundaries in ways that are inappropriate or uncomfortable.

In a digital age where personal information is readily accessible, the invasion of privacy has taken on new dimensions. The unauthorized access to someone's emails, social media accounts, or personal devices constitutes a breach of trust and honesty. It not only violates their privacy but also demonstrates a lack of respect for their boundaries.

In relationships, whether personal or professional, it's essential to establish and respect boundaries. Open and honest communication about what is considered private and what can be shared is crucial. Trust is fostered when individuals feel that their boundaries are being respected, and their privacy is valued.

In conclusion, trust and honesty are invaluable in any relationship, and they are often interdependent. Consistent dishonesty or omissions, trust-breaking behavior, and privacy invasion can all serve to undermine these vital foundations. Rebuilding trust after it has been damaged is challenging but not impossible, requiring sincere effort, time, and a commitment to change. Ultimately, nurturing trust and honesty in our interactions with others is essential for maintaining healthy and meaningful connections in our lives.

CHAPTER 4

Respect and Boundaries

4.1 Disregard for Personal Boundaries

4.2 Verbal or Physical Abuse

4.3 Lack of Respect for Your Opinions and Feelings

Respect and boundaries are two fundamental pillars upon which healthy relationships are built. They serve as the bedrock of mutual understanding, trust, and emotional well-being. In this discussion, we will delve into the importance of respect and the consequences of disregarding personal boundaries. We will also explore the damaging effects of verbal or physical abuse and the significance of respecting each other's opinions and feelings.

4.1 Disregard for Personal Boundaries

Personal boundaries define the limits we set to protect our physical, emotional, and mental well-being. They establish the space in which we feel safe and comfortable. Disregarding these boundaries can lead to severe consequences in any relationship, be it romantic, familial, or professional.

When someone disregards your personal boundaries, it can manifest in various ways. It could be a partner who invades your personal space without permission, a friend who constantly disrespects your need for alone time, or a colleague who oversteps their professional boundaries by prying into your personal life. Regardless of the context, the message is clear: your comfort and autonomy are being violated.

The consequences of such disregard can be damaging. It erodes trust and can lead to feelings of resentment, anxiety, and vulnerability. Over time, if personal boundaries continue to be disregarded, it can even result in the breakdown of the relationship altogether. It is essential for individuals to recognize and respect each other's boundaries to ensure a healthy and harmonious connection.

4.2 Verbal or Physical Abuse

Verbal and physical abuse represent the most extreme forms of disrespect within a relationship. These actions not only cross boundaries but trample upon the very essence of respect. Verbal abuse encompasses hurtful words, insults, degradation, and threats, while physical abuse involves any form of physical harm or violence.

The consequences of abuse are profound and far-reaching. Victims often suffer not only physically but emotionally as well. They may experience feelings of worthlessness, fear, and depression. The trauma inflicted by abuse can have lasting effects, leading to a cycle of pain that is difficult to break.

It is crucial to recognize that abuse is never acceptable, and it is never the fault of the victim. Building and maintaining healthy relationships requires a commitment to treating each other with kindness, empathy, and respect. If you or someone you know is experiencing abuse, seeking help from a counselor, therapist, or support network is essential to breaking free from this cycle and rebuilding one's life with the respect and dignity deserved.

4.3 Lack of Respect for Your Opinions and Feelings

Respecting someone's opinions and feelings is a fundamental aspect of showing respect in any relationship. It means valuing their thoughts, beliefs, and emotions, even when they differ from your own. When this respect is absent, it can lead to communication breakdowns, hurt feelings, and a sense of invalidation.

In a healthy relationship, individuals should feel free to express themselves without fear of judgment or dismissal. They should be able to voice their opinions and share their feelings without the fear of being ridiculed or ignored. When respect for each other's viewpoints and emotions is present, it fosters open and honest communication, strengthening the bond between individuals.

Conversely, when this respect is lacking, it can lead to frustration and resentment. Feelings of being unheard or unimportant can cause emotional distance and conflict. Over time, the absence of respect for each other's opinions and feelings can erode the foundation of the relationship.

In conclusion, respect and boundaries are non-negotiable elements of healthy relationships. Disregard for personal boundaries, whether through physical intrusion or emotional manipulation, can have detrimental effects on trust and well-being. Verbal and physical abuse represent the darkest extremes of disrespect, causing profound harm to victims. Furthermore, a lack of respect for each other's opinions and feelings can lead to communication breakdowns and emotional distance.

It is essential for individuals to understand the importance of respect and boundaries and actively work towards maintaining them in all their relationships. By doing so, they can create a nurturing and supportive environment where each person's autonomy and feelings are valued, fostering strong, enduring connections built on trust and empathy.

CHAPTER 5

Time and Prioritization

5.1 Consistently Putting Others Before You

5.2 Neglecting Quality Time Together

5.3 Frequent Canceling of Plans

Time is a precious commodity that often seems to slip through our fingers faster than we can grasp it. In today's fast-paced world, the allocation of time and prioritization has become an art form, especially in the context of relationships. This essay will delve into three key aspects of time and prioritization within relationships: consistently putting others before you, neglecting quality time together, and frequent canceling of plans.

5.1 Consistently Putting Others Before You

One common pitfall in relationships is the tendency to consistently put others before oneself. While selflessness is a virtue, it can become detrimental when it becomes a pattern. People often prioritize the needs and desires of their partners, friends, or family members over their own, believing that this self-sacrifice is a sign of love and devotion. However, this can lead to feelings of resentment and burnout over time.

When individuals consistently put others before themselves, they risk neglecting their own well-being. They may sacrifice their own goals, passions, and self-care in the process. Over time, this can lead to feelings of frustration and imbalance within the relationship. It's essential to strike a balance between giving to others and taking care of oneself. Prioritizing self-care, setting boundaries, and communicating openly with loved ones can help create a healthier dynamic.

5.2 Neglecting Quality Time Together

Quality time is the cornerstone of any meaningful relationship. However, in our increasingly busy lives, it's easy to neglect this crucial aspect of connection. Neglecting quality time together can erode the foundation of a relationship, leading to feelings of distance and emotional disconnection.

Many people fall into the trap of substituting quantity for quality when it comes to spending time with their loved ones. They may be physically present but mentally absent, distracted by work, technology, or other commitments. This can lead to partners or family members feeling undervalued and unimportant.

To address this issue, individuals must prioritize genuine quality time with their loved ones. This means setting aside distractions, actively listening, and engaging in meaningful activities that foster connection. Regular date nights, unplugged weekends, or simply being fully present during conversations can rekindle the emotional bond between individuals and strengthen their relationships.

5.3 Frequent Canceling of Plans

The frequent canceling of plans is a behavior that can wreak havoc on relationships. Whether it's canceling a dinner date with a friend, backing out of a commitment to a partner, or neglecting plans with family members, this habit sends a message that one's time is not valued. It can lead to hurt feelings, disappointment, and a breakdown of trust.

There are various reasons why people cancel plans, ranging from work-related emergencies to feeling overwhelmed by social commitments. However, it's essential to strike a balance between honoring one's commitments and acknowledging personal limitations. Consistently canceling plans without valid reasons can strain relationships and lead to a lack of reliability.

To address this issue, individuals must communicate honestly with their loved ones. If they find themselves frequently canceling plans, it's important to explain the reasons and express remorse for any inconvenience caused. Moreover, striving to prioritize commitments and manage time more effectively can help reduce the need to cancel plans regularly.

In conclusion, time and prioritization are pivotal aspects of maintaining healthy and fulfilling relationships. Consistently putting others before oneself, neglecting quality time together, and frequently canceling plans are all behaviors that can undermine the bonds between individuals. To build and sustain meaningful connections, it's crucial to strike a balance between self-care and caring for others, prioritize quality over quantity when spending time together, and uphold commitments and reliability. By addressing these aspects of time and prioritization, individuals can nurture stronger, more resilient relationships in an increasingly fast-paced world.

CHAPTER 6

Emotional Well-being

6.1 Emotional Manipulation

6.2 Gaslighting

6.3 Constant Criticism or Belittling

Emotional well-being is a fundamental component of Emotional Well-being: Navigating the Shadows of Manipulation, Gaslighting, and Criticism

Emotional well-being is a fundamental component of our overall health and happiness. It encompasses our ability to understand, express, and manage our emotions in a healthy way. Unfortunately, in today's complex world, emotional well-being can be challenged by various negative influences, including emotional manipulation, gaslighting, and constant criticism or belittling.

6.1 Emotional Manipulation

Emotional manipulation is a tactic used by individuals to control or influence the emotions, thoughts, and behaviors of others for their own benefit. It often involves subtle, coercive, or deceptive tactics that can be difficult to detect. This form of manipulation can take many forms, from passive-aggressive comments to guilt-tripping or playing the victim.

One common aspect of emotional manipulation is guilt-tripping. Manipulators use guilt to make their targets feel responsible for their actions or decisions. They may say things like, "If you really cared about me, you would do this for me." Over time, this constant guilt-tripping can erode a person's self-esteem and self-worth, leading to emotional distress.

Another aspect of emotional manipulation is gaslighting, which we'll explore further in the next section. Emotional manipulation can also include tactics like withholding affection or giving the silent treatment to control someone's behavior. All of these tactics can cause significant harm to an individual's emotional well-being.

To protect oneself from emotional manipulation, it's crucial to recognize the signs. These may include feeling constantly guilty or responsible for someone else's feelings, experiencing anxiety or depression in a specific relationship, or noticing that your emotions and actions are consistently controlled by someone else. Setting boundaries and seeking support from trusted friends or professionals can help break free from emotional manipulation's grip.

6.2 Gaslighting

Gaslighting is a particularly insidious form of emotional manipulation that involves manipulating someone into doubting their own perceptions, memory, or sanity. The term originates from a play and later a film called "Gas Light," in which a husband tries to convince his wife that she's going insane by dimming the gas lights but denying it.

Gaslighting can be devastating to an individual's emotional well-being. It often involves the gaslighter denying that they said or did something hurtful, even when there is concrete evidence to the contrary. They may tell their target that they're "too sensitive" or "imagining things." Over time, this relentless denial can lead the victim to question their own reality and lose confidence in their judgment.

Victims of gaslighting may experience anxiety, depression, and a deep sense of confusion. They may feel trapped in a reality that the gaslighter has constructed for them, one where their emotions and perceptions are constantly invalidated.

Recognizing gaslighting is the first step to protecting oneself from its harm. Trusting your own feelings and perceptions is essential. Keeping a journal or record of interactions with the gaslighter can provide evidence of their manipulation. Seeking support from a therapist or counselor can also be invaluable in regaining one's emotional well-being after experiencing gaslighting.

6.3 Constant Criticism or Belittling

Constant criticism or belittling is a form of emotional abuse that can gradually chip away at a person's self-esteem and emotional well-being. This type of abuse often takes place in personal relationships, such as romantic partnerships or within families, but it can also occur in professional settings.

Criticism is a normal part of life, and constructive feedback can help us grow and improve. However, constant criticism that is intended to demean or belittle is harmful. It can manifest as name-calling, insults, mockery, or nitpicking. Over time, the person subjected to such treatment may begin to internalize these negative messages, leading to feelings of worthlessness and inadequacy.

Belittling can also take the form of minimizing someone's achievements or making them feel inferior. It's often used as a way for the abuser to exert control and maintain power in the relationship. This constant erosion of a person's self-esteem can have long-lasting effects on their emotional well-being, leading to issues like anxiety, depression, and low self-confidence.

Recognizing the signs of constant criticism or belittling is vital for one's emotional well-being. If you find yourself in a relationship where you are constantly subjected to these behaviors, seeking support from a therapist or counselor can provide guidance on setting boundaries and developing strategies to protect your self-esteem.

In conclusion, emotional well-being is a precious aspect of our lives that should be nurtured and protected. Recognizing and addressing emotional manipulation, gaslighting, and constant criticism or belittling is essential for maintaining a healthy emotional state. Seeking support from trusted individuals or professionals can be a crucial step toward reclaiming one's emotional well-being and building resilience against these harmful influences. Remember, you deserve to be in relationships that uplift and support your emotional health. our overall health and happiness. It encompasses our ability to understand, express, and manage our emotions in a healthy way. Unfortunately, in today's complex world, emotional well-being can be challenged by various negative influences, including emotional manipulation, gaslighting, and constant criticism or belittling.

CHAPTER 7

Financial Compatibility

7.1 Financial Secrets or Irresponsible Behavior

7.2 Incompatible Financial Goals

Money is a fundamental aspect of our lives, and it plays a pivotal role in our relationships. Financial compatibility, or the lack thereof, can significantly impact the health and longevity of a partnership. In this exploration, we delve into two crucial aspects of financial compatibility: financial secrets and incompatible financial goals.

7.1 Financial Secrets or Irresponsible Behavior

Honesty is often touted as the cornerstone of any successful relationship, and this principle applies with particular vigor to financial matters. Financial secrets, whether they stem from undisclosed debt, hidden income, or secret expenditures, can erode trust and breed resentment. In some cases, these secrets may manifest as irresponsible financial behavior, like compulsive spending or reckless investing.

Financial secrets often arise from fear - fear of judgment, fear of conflict, or fear of upsetting the delicate balance of a relationship. However, these secrets have a way of unraveling over time, causing deeper wounds than the initial fear sought to avoid.

Consider a scenario where one partner discovers that the other has been hiding significant credit card debt. The sense of betrayal and deception can be devastating. This breach of trust can lead to arguments, emotional distance, and, in the worst cases, dissolution of the relationship.

The key to addressing financial secrets or irresponsible behavior lies in open and non-judgmental communication. Couples must create a safe space where they can honestly discuss their financial situations and mistakes. This dialogue should be focused on understanding and supporting each other rather than assigning blame.

In some cases, professional financial counseling or therapy may be necessary to address underlying issues that contribute to financial secrets or irresponsible behavior. The goal is not just to mend the financial wounds but also to strengthen the emotional bond between partners.

7.2 Incompatible Financial Goals

Financial compatibility also hinges on having compatible financial goals and priorities. While individual financial goals can vary widely, it's crucial that a couple's goals align sufficiently for a harmonious partnership.

Consider a couple where one partner dreams of early retirement and extensive travel while the other is focused on buying a home and starting a family. These goals, while not inherently conflicting, can strain a relationship if not addressed and harmonized.

Incompatibility in financial goals can lead to constant arguments and disagreements about how to allocate resources. One partner may feel resentful if they perceive that their financial aspirations are being sacrificed for the other's dreams. This discord can fester and damage the relationship over time.

To address incompatible financial goals, couples should engage in open and constructive discussions about their long-term objectives. Compromise is often necessary, as it's unlikely that two individuals will have identical financial aspirations. Finding common ground and crafting a shared vision for the future can help bridge these differences.

It's also essential to recognize that financial goals can evolve over time. Couples should revisit their financial plans periodically to ensure that they remain aligned with their changing circumstances and desires. This flexibility can prevent conflicts that arise from rigidly clinging to outdated goals.

In some cases, it may be beneficial to involve a financial planner or advisor who can provide objective guidance and help couples chart a path towards their shared financial objectives. This outside perspective can be invaluable in navigating the complexities of merging financial lives.

In conclusion, financial compatibility is a vital component of a successful and enduring relationship. Financial secrets or irresponsible behavior can corrode trust and intimacy, while incompatible financial goals can lead to ongoing conflict. The key to addressing these challenges lies in open communication, understanding, and compromise. Couples who can navigate these financial waters together are more likely to build a strong and lasting partnership based on trust and shared aspirations.

CHAPTER 8

Intimacy and Affection

8.1 Lack of Intimacy or Affection

8.2 Withholding Affection as a Punishment

8.3 Incompatibility in Sexual Preferences or Frequency

Intimacy and affection are vital components of any healthy and fulfilling relationship. These elements foster emotional connection, trust, and overall satisfaction between partners. However, like any aspect of a relationship, intimacy and affection can face challenges. In this exploration, we will delve into three key aspects: the lack of intimacy or affection, withholding affection as a punishment, and incompatibility in sexual preferences or frequency.

8.1 Lack of Intimacy or Affection

The absence of intimacy or affection in a relationship can be deeply distressing. Intimacy encompasses both physical and emotional closeness, while affection involves expressing love and care through actions and words. When these elements are lacking, it can lead to feelings of loneliness, dissatisfaction, and even resentment.

Several factors can contribute to a lack of intimacy or affection. Stress, busy schedules, and external pressures can all take a toll on a couple's ability to connect on an intimate level. Additionally, past traumas or unresolved issues may create emotional barriers that hinder the development of intimacy. Communication breakdowns can also play a significant role; partners might not understand each other's needs or may fear vulnerability.

Addressing a lack of intimacy or affection requires open and honest communication. Couples should create a safe space to discuss their feelings and desires. Seeking professional help, such as couples therapy, can be instrumental in identifying underlying issues and developing strategies to rebuild intimacy.

8.2 Withholding Affection as a Punishment

Using affection as a weapon to punish a partner is a toxic behavior that can erode trust and the foundation of a relationship. This manipulation tactic often stems from unresolved conflicts or a desire for power and control. When one partner withholds affection, it creates a hostile and emotionally damaging environment.

Withholding affection can take various forms, including physical distance, silent treatment, or even engaging in passive-aggressive behavior. These actions send a clear message of rejection and can leave the other partner feeling hurt, unloved, and confused.

To address this issue, both partners must be willing to recognize and confront the problem. The person withholding affection needs to explore the reasons behind their behavior and work on healthier ways to express their feelings or resolve conflicts. The recipient of this behavior should assert their boundaries and communicate their needs for a loving and respectful relationship. In many cases, couples therapy can help address these issues and promote healthier patterns of interaction.

8.3 Incompatibility in Sexual Preferences or Frequency

Sexual compatibility is an essential aspect of intimacy in a romantic relationship. It involves the alignment of both partners' sexual desires, preferences, and frequency of engagement. When there is a significant gap in this aspect of a relationship, it can lead to dissatisfaction and potential conflicts.

Incompatibility in sexual preferences may involve differences in desires, fantasies, or even boundaries. For example, one partner may have a higher sex drive than the other, or they may have varying interests in sexual activities. These differences can create frustration and resentment if not addressed openly.

Addressing sexual incompatibility requires sensitivity, communication, and compromise. Partners should engage in honest conversations about their desires and boundaries. It's essential to create an environment where both individuals feel safe expressing their needs without judgment. Exploring new ways to connect physically and emotionally can also be beneficial.

If sexual incompatibility persists despite efforts to resolve it, seeking guidance from a sex therapist or counselor can be a valuable step. These professionals can help couples navigate the complexities of their sexual relationship and find solutions that work for both partners.

In conclusion, intimacy and affection are the bedrock of healthy and fulfilling relationships. Their absence or mismanagement can lead to a breakdown in trust and satisfaction. However, with open communication, empathy, and a willingness to address issues head-on, couples can overcome challenges related to the lack of intimacy or affection, the use of affection as a punishment, and incompatibility in sexual preferences or frequency. By prioritizing these aspects of their relationship, couples can build stronger bonds and experience greater happiness together.

CHAPTER 9

Social and Family Relationships

9.1 Isolation from Friends and Family

9.2 Constant Conflict with Loved Ones

9.3 Clashes in Values and Beliefs

Social and family relationships are the cornerstones of human life, providing a sense of belonging, support, and connection. However, these relationships can also be fraught with challenges, leading to isolation, conflict, and clashes in values and beliefs. This essay explores these three aspects of social and family relationships, shedding light on the dynamics that can either strengthen or strain these vital connections.

9.1 Isolation from Friends and Family

Isolation from friends and family members can be a distressing experience that has profound effects on one's emotional well-being. Various factors can contribute to this sense of isolation, from geographical distance to personal conflicts or external circumstances. One common cause of isolation is the fast-paced, digitally-driven world we live in. As individuals become increasingly engrossed in their online lives, physical interactions with loved ones can take a backseat. The convenience of virtual communication can inadvertently lead to a sense of detachment from the real world.

Moreover, life transitions such as relocation for work or education can result in physical separation from one's established support network. While these changes may offer exciting opportunities, they can also create feelings of loneliness and isolation, particularly when individuals struggle to establish new connections in unfamiliar environments.

Additionally, the digital age has brought about new challenges in maintaining close relationships. The allure of social media can sometimes create a false sense of connection. People may have hundreds of online "friends" and followers, yet still feel profoundly isolated. The superficiality of many online interactions can exacerbate feelings of loneliness as individuals yearn for more meaningful, face-to-face connections.

To mitigate isolation from friends and family, it's crucial to prioritize these relationships. Actively seeking out opportunities for in-person interactions, even in a world dominated by screens, can help bridge the gap. Open communication about feelings of isolation can also be a crucial step in reconnecting with loved ones.

9.2 Constant Conflict with Loved Ones

Conflict is a natural part of any relationship, but when it becomes constant, it can be detrimental. Constant conflict with loved ones can take a significant toll on one's emotional and mental health. The sources of conflict in family and social relationships are diverse, ranging from differences in communication styles to unresolved past issues or clashing personalities.

One common trigger of constant conflict is miscommunication. People often have varying ways of expressing themselves, and misunderstanding or misinterpretation can escalate minor disagreements into major battles. Furthermore, unresolved issues from the past can linger beneath the surface, erupting into conflicts when triggered by seemingly unrelated events.

Another factor contributing to constant conflict is personality differences. In close relationships, individuals may have vastly different temperaments and coping mechanisms. These differences can lead to frequent disagreements and misunderstandings if not addressed and managed effectively.

The impact of constant conflict on mental health cannot be overstated. It can lead to anxiety, depression, and a diminished sense of self-worth. Prolonged conflict can erode trust and intimacy, making it difficult to repair the damage done to the relationship.

To address constant conflict with loved ones, it's essential to develop effective communication skills. This includes active listening, empathy, and the ability to express one's needs and feelings clearly. Seeking professional help, such as couples therapy or family counseling, can also be beneficial in resolving deeply rooted conflicts and rebuilding relationships.

9.3 Clashes in Values and Beliefs

Clashes in values and beliefs are another significant challenge that can strain social and family relationships. Our values and beliefs shape our worldview, influencing our decisions, priorities, and behaviors. When individuals within a family or social group hold divergent values and beliefs, it can lead to tension and conflict.

Clashes in values often become most apparent in areas such as religion, politics, and ethics. These are deeply personal and emotionally charged topics, and disagreements can quickly escalate. For example, a person with strong environmentalist beliefs may clash with a family member who prioritizes economic growth over environmental conservation.

These clashes can be particularly challenging because they touch on fundamental aspects of a person's identity. When individuals feel that their core values are being invalidated or disrespected, it can lead to feelings of anger, frustration, and alienation.

However, it's important to recognize that diversity of thought and belief is a natural part of the human experience. Embracing these differences can lead to personal growth and richer, more robust relationships. To navigate clashes in values and beliefs, open and respectful dialogue is essential. This means actively listening to others' perspectives, seeking common ground, and agreeing to disagree when necessary.

Conclusion

Social and family relationships are integral to our well-being, but they are not immune to challenges. Isolation from friends and family, constant conflict with loved ones, and clashes in values and beliefs are all aspects of human relationships that can test our resilience and patience.

Addressing these challenges requires self-awareness, empathy, and effective communication. It's important to prioritize meaningful, in-person connections in an increasingly digital world, manage conflicts with loved ones through healthy communication strategies, and navigate clashes in values and beliefs with an open and respectful mindset.

Ultimately, nurturing and sustaining social and family relationships is an ongoing journey that requires effort and understanding from all parties involved. By recognizing and addressing these challenges, we can cultivate stronger, more fulfilling connections with the people who matter most in our lives.

CHAPTER 10

Recognizing Patterns

10.1 Identifying Repeated Red Flags

10.2 Understanding the Cycle of Abuse

Patterns are an inherent part of human existence. From the rhythmic cycles of day and night to the predictable sequences of seasons, our lives are governed by patterns. Patterns offer us a sense of stability and predictability in an otherwise chaotic world. However, not all patterns are benign; some can be deeply troubling and harmful. In this discussion, we delve into the realm of recognizing patterns, specifically in two critical contexts: identifying repeated red flags and understanding the cycle of abuse.

10.1: Identifying Repeated Red Flags

When it comes to personal relationships and decision-making, recognizing repeated red flags is a skill that can make a significant difference in one's life. Red flags are warning signs or indicators of potential problems, and when they repeat, they become patterns that demand our attention.

1. Relationship Red Flags

In the realm of personal relationships, red flags can manifest in various ways. These warning signs often include consistent behaviors or attitudes that signal potential issues. Some common relationship red flags include:

-Lack of Communication: Repeatedly avoiding open and honest communication can be a significant red flag. Healthy relationships thrive on communication and mutual understanding.

-Unhealthy Jealousy: When one partner consistently displays excessive jealousy or possessiveness, it can be a sign of insecurity or controlling tendencies.

Disrespect: Repeated instances of disrespect, whether it's name-calling, belittling, or undermining, can be an alarming pattern that may lead to emotional abuse.

-Isolation: If someone tries to isolate you from friends and family on a consistent basis, it could be a sign of coercive control or manipulation.

2. Professional Red Flags

Recognizing patterns of repeated red flags is also crucial in the professional sphere. These flags can help us make informed decisions about our career paths and workplace environments. Some common professional red flags include:

-High Turnover Rates: Companies with a history of frequent employee turnover may have underlying issues, such as a toxic work culture or poor management.

-Lack of Accountability: If a company consistently fails to take responsibility for its mistakes or address employee concerns, it could indicate a problematic pattern of behavior.

-Ethical Concerns: Repeated ethical violations within a company should not be ignored. Consistent disregard for ethical standards can lead to legal and reputational issues.

-Inadequate Work-Life Balance: A pattern of overworking employees and disregarding work-life balance can negatively impact well-being and job satisfaction.

3. Financial Red Flags

In the realm of personal finance, identifying patterns of repeated red flags is crucial for long-term financial health. These financial red flags often involve recurring behaviors that can lead to financial instability or crisis. Some common financial red flags include:

-Consistent Overspending: Repeatedly spending beyond one's means or accumulating debt without a clear plan for repayment is a significant red flag.

- **Ignoring Savings**: Consistently neglecting to save money for emergencies or long-term goals can lead to financial vulnerability.

-Avoiding Financial Discussions: If a partner or family member consistently avoids discussing financial matters, it may indicate financial secrets or mismanagement.

-Pattern of Impulsive Purchases: Frequent, impulsive purchases without consideration of their long-term impact on finances can signal a lack of financial responsibility.

Recognizing these repeated red flags in various aspects of life can empower individuals to make informed decisions, whether it's about relationships, careers, or finances. It's important to remember that patterns of red flags are not to be taken lightly and often warrant further investigation or intervention.

10.2 : Understanding the Cycle of Abuse

The cycle of abuse is a deeply troubling and harmful pattern that occurs in abusive relationships. It's essential to understand this cycle to break free from it or to help those who may be trapped in it.

1. The Tension-Building Phase

The cycle of abuse typically begins with the tension-building phase. During this period, minor conflicts and disagreements escalate, and the victim often feels the need to walk on eggshells to avoid triggering the abuser's anger. Communication deteriorates, and tension in the relationship intensifies. The victim may resort to appeasing the abuser to keep the peace.

2. The Explosive Phase

The tension eventually reaches a breaking point, leading to the explosive phase. In this stage, the abuser's anger and aggression escalate dramatically. Verbal, emotional, or physical abuse occurs, leaving the victim traumatized and in fear for their safety. This phase can lead to severe harm, both physically and psychologically.

3. The Honeymoon Phase

Following the explosive phase, the abuser often enters the honeymoon phase. During this stage, they may express remorse, apologize profusely, and promise to change their behavior. They may shower the victim with affection, gifts, or gestures of love, creating a false sense of security and hope that the abuse will stop.

4. The Reconciliation Phase

The reconciliation phase is marked by the victim's willingness to forgive and believe the abuser's promises of change. This hope for a better future keeps the victim trapped in the cycle, as they desperately want the relationship to improve. However, this phase is often short-lived, as the cycle of abuse repeats itself.

Understanding the cycle of abuse is crucial because it highlights the manipulative and cyclical nature of abusive relationships. Victims may feel trapped by the repeated pattern of tension, abuse, false apologies, and hope for change. Breaking free from this cycle often requires support from friends, family, or professional help.

In conclusion, recognizing patterns, whether they involve identifying repeated red flags or understanding the cycle of abuse, is a vital life skill. These patterns can significantly impact our personal relationships, professional lives, and financial well-being. By honing our ability to identify and respond to these patterns, we empower ourselves to make informed decisions and create healthier, more fulfilling lives. It is crucial to remember that recognizing patterns is not enough; taking appropriate action when red flags appear or when abuse is identified is equally essential for personal growth and well-being.

CHAPTER 11

Self-Reflection

11.1 Assessing Your Own Role in the Relationship

11.2 Recognizing Your Own Boundaries and Needs

Self-reflection is a powerful tool that allows individuals to gain insight into themselves, their actions, and their relationships. In this exploration of self-reflection, we will delve into two critical aspects: assessing your own role in a relationship and recognizing your own boundaries and needs. These two components are essential for personal growth and the development of healthier, more fulfilling connections with others.

Assessing Your Own Role in the Relationship

Relationships, whether they are personal or professional, are intricate and multifaceted. Often, when things go awry, individuals tend to point fingers and assign blame to the other party involved. However, a fundamental aspect of self-reflection involves taking a step back and assessing one's own role in the relationship dynamics.

1. Self-Awareness: The first step in assessing your role in a relationship is to cultivate self-awareness. This means being honest with yourself about your thoughts, feelings, and actions within the relationship. Ask yourself questions like, "How do I contribute to the dynamics of this relationship? What are my strengths and weaknesses in relating to this person?"

2. Empathy: Empathy plays a crucial role in understanding your impact on others. Try to put yourself in the other person's shoes and consider how your words and actions might have affected them. Were there times when you could have been more sensitive or understanding?

3. Communication: Effective communication is vital for assessing your role in a relationship. Engage in open and honest conversations with the other person to gain their perspective.

Sometimes, misunderstandings can be cleared up through dialogue, leading to better mutual understanding.

4. Patterns of Behavior: Reflect on any recurring patterns of behavior in your relationships. Do you tend to react in similar ways in various situations? Recognizing these patterns can help you identify areas for personal growth and change.

5. Responsibility: Accepting responsibility for your actions is a hallmark of self-reflection. Acknowledge any mistakes or shortcomings on your part, and be willing to make amends or improvements where necessary.

6. Feedback: Seek feedback from trusted friends, family members, or mentors. They can provide valuable insights into your behavior and its impact on others. Sometimes, an outside perspective can reveal blind spots you might have missed.

7. Goal Setting: Once you've assessed your role in a relationship, set specific goals for improvement. These goals should be realistic and actionable, such as working on active listening, managing your emotions better, or being more supportive.

Recognizing Your Own Boundaries and Needs

Healthy relationships are built on a foundation of mutual respect for each other's boundaries and needs. It's essential to recognize and communicate your own boundaries and needs effectively. Here's how self-reflection can help in this regard:

1. Self-Exploration: Begin by delving into your own inner world. What are your values, beliefs, and priorities? What makes you feel comfortable, and what are your limits in a relationship?

2. **Boundaries**: Boundaries are the invisible lines that define what is acceptable and unacceptable in a relationship. Reflect on what your boundaries are in various aspects of your life, such as personal space, emotional sharing, and time management.

3. **Needs**: Consider your emotional, physical, and psychological needs in a relationship. What do you require to feel supported and fulfilled? Understanding your needs is crucial for finding compatibility with others.

4. **Communication**: Once you've identified your boundaries and needs, communicate them clearly and assertively to the people in your life. Effective communication ensures that your

expectations are understood, reducing the likelihood of misunderstandings.

5. **Respect for Others' Boundaries and Needs**: Just as you expect others to respect your boundaries and needs, reciprocate by respecting theirs. Self-reflection can help you develop empathy and understanding for the boundaries and needs of others.

6. **Adaptability**: Be open to negotiation and compromise in relationships. Sometimes, your boundaries and needs may need to adjust to accommodate the needs of others, and vice versa. Self-reflection can help you navigate these situations with maturity.

7. **Reevaluation**: Periodically revisit your boundaries and needs as circumstances change. What was acceptable in one phase of your life may evolve over time. Regular self-reflection ensures that your expectations align with your current reality.

In conclusion, self-reflection is a powerful tool for personal growth and for building healthier, more meaningful relationships. Assessing your own role in a relationship and recognizing your own boundaries and needs are integral aspects of this process. By cultivating self-awareness, empathy, effective communication, and a willingness to adapt, you can nurture more fulfilling and harmonious connections with others. Self-reflection is not a one-time exercise but a lifelong journey towards greater self-understanding and better relationships.

CHAPTER 12

Seeking Help and Support

12.1 Talking to Friends and Family

12.2 Considering Professional Help

Seeking Help and Support: A Path to Healing and Growth

Life is a complex journey, filled with its share of challenges, triumphs, and everything in between. During these various phases of life, there are moments when seeking help and support becomes not just an option but a necessity. In this exploration of the topic, we will delve into two critical aspects of seeking help and support: talking to friends and family and considering professional help. These avenues provide vital resources for individuals to navigate the ups and downs of life.

Talking to Friends and Family

Friends and family are often our closest allies in times of need. They can provide emotional support, a listening ear, and valuable insights into our situations. Here are some key points to consider when seeking help and support from friends and family:

1. Trust and Vulnerability: Opening up to friends and family requires trust and vulnerability. It can be challenging to share our innermost thoughts and feelings, but doing so can lead to a deeper connection and understanding between individuals.

2. Active Listening: When talking to friends and family, it's essential to practice active listening. This means giving the person your full attention, asking clarifying questions, and refraining from judgment or interruption. By being present in the conversation, you show that you value their perspective.

3. Empathy and Validation: Friends and family can offer empathy and validation for your experiences. Validation acknowledges your feelings as valid and helps you feel understood. Empathy goes a step further, as it involves genuinely understanding and sharing in another person's feelings.

4. Perspective and Advice: Friends and family can offer different perspectives on your situation. They might provide advice, share their own experiences, or offer solutions you hadn't considered. However, remember that their advice is based on their own perspectives and may not always align with your needs.

5. Boundaries: While seeking support from loved ones, it's essential to respect boundaries. Some individuals may not be comfortable discussing certain topics or may need space. It's crucial to honor their boundaries and communicate your own as well.

6. Reciprocity: Supporting one another is a two-way street. Just as you seek help and support from friends and family, be ready to reciprocate when they need assistance. Building a network of mutual support strengthens relationships and creates a sense of community.

7. Time and Patience: Understand that not everyone will respond to your needs in the same way or at the same speed. Give your loved ones the time and space they need to process your request for help and support.

Considering Professional Help

While friends and family are invaluable sources of support, there are situations where seeking professional help becomes essential for personal growth, healing, and well-being. Professional help can come in various forms, including therapists, counselors, doctors, and coaches. Here are some important points to consider when thinking about professional help:

1. Specialized Expertise: Professionals bring specialized knowledge and expertise to the table. Therapists, for example, are trained to address mental and emotional health concerns, while doctors can provide medical solutions. Seeking professional help ensures that you receive the most appropriate guidance for your specific situation.

2. Confidentiality: Professional help often comes with a high degree of confidentiality. This means you can speak openly about your concerns without fear of judgment or your information being shared with others.

3. Objective Perspective: Professionals provide an objective perspective. They are not emotionally invested in your situation, allowing them to offer unbiased insights and guidance.

4. Tools and Techniques: Professionals often use evidence-based tools and techniques to help individuals overcome challenges. Whether it's cognitive-behavioral therapy, medication, or other therapeutic methods, these approaches can be highly effective in promoting personal growth and recovery.

5. Safe Space: Therapy and counseling sessions provide a safe and supportive space to explore your thoughts, emotions, and behaviors. This can be especially beneficial for addressing issues like trauma, addiction, or complex emotional struggles.

6. Crisis Intervention: In times of crisis or acute distress, professional help can be a lifeline. Immediate intervention by a mental health professional or medical expert can be critical in such situations.

7. Long-term Growth: Professional help is not limited to crisis intervention; it can also be a valuable resource for long-term personal growth. Therapy, for instance, can help individuals develop coping strategies, improve relationships, and work through deep-seated issues.

8. Self-Care: Seeking professional help is a form of self-care. It demonstrates a commitment to your well-being and personal development. It's a proactive step towards addressing challenges and improving the quality of your life.

9. Accessibility: Professional help is often more accessible than ever before. Telehealth and online counseling options have expanded access to mental health services, making it easier for individuals to connect with professionals.

10. No Shame in Seeking Help: There is no shame in seeking professional help. Mental health struggles, emotional challenges, and personal issues are part of the human experience. Seeking help is a sign of strength, not weakness.

In conclusion, seeking help and support is a fundamental aspect of human existence. It encompasses reaching out to friends and family for emotional support, empathy, and validation, as well as considering professional help when facing complex or enduring challenges. Both avenues have their unique benefits and can be vital in fostering personal growth, healing, and well-being. The key is recognizing when to lean on each of these sources and being proactive in seeking the support you need. Ultimately, seeking help and support is a courageous and empowering choice that can lead to greater resilience and a more fulfilling life.

CHAPTER 13

Making Decisions

13.1 Evaluating the Relationship

13.2 Exploring Options: Repair, Improve, or Leave

Making decisions is an integral part of human life. From the moment we wake up to the time we go to bed, we are faced with choices that shape our day, our relationships, and our future. Some decisions are small, like choosing what to have for breakfast, while others are significant, like deciding on a career path or whether to end a long-term relationship. In this essay, we will delve into the process of making decisions, focusing on two key aspects:

evaluating the relationship and exploring options—specifically, whether to repair, improve, or leave.

Evaluating the Relationship

The first step in making any decision is to evaluate the current situation or relationship. Whether it's a personal or professional context, understanding the dynamics at play is crucial. When it comes to evaluating a relationship, there are several key factors to consider:

1. Communication: Effective communication is the cornerstone of any healthy relationship. Assess how well you and the other party communicate. Are there open lines of communication, or do issues often go unaddressed?

2. Trust: Trust is the foundation of any successful relationship. Evaluate whether trust exists and if it has been compromised in any way. Trust can be eroded by lies, deceit, or broken promises.

3. Compatibility: Consider whether you and the other person are fundamentally compatible in terms of values, goals, and interests. Compatibility can greatly influence the long-term viability of a relationship.

4. Respect: Mutual respect is vital. Do both parties respect each other's boundaries, opinions, and feelings? Respect forms the basis for a healthy and harmonious relationship.

5. Emotional Well-being: Assess how the relationship affects your emotional well-being. Do you feel happy, supported, and secure, or is it a source of stress and negativity?

6. Conflict Resolution: Evaluate how conflicts are handled within the relationship. Are disagreements resolved constructively, or do they escalate into destructive arguments?

7. Future Goals: Consider whether both parties share similar long-term goals and visions for the relationship. Misalignment in future aspirations can create significant challenges.

8. Red Flags: Pay attention to any red flags or warning signs, such as abusive behavior, manipulation, or a consistent lack of effort from the other party.

Taking the time to thoroughly assess these aspects of a relationship can provide valuable insights into its overall health and whether it's worth investing in. However, evaluating a relationship is only the first step. Once you have a clear understanding of where things stand, the next crucial step is exploring your options.

Exploring Options: Repair, Improve, or Leave

When faced with a relationship that requires attention, you have three primary options: repair, improve, or leave. The choice you make depends on the specific circumstances and the potential for positive change.

1. Repair

Repairing a relationship involves addressing and resolving existing issues to restore its health and vitality. This option is ideal when both parties are committed to making the necessary changes and working together to overcome challenges. Repairing a relationship often requires:

- Open Communication: Start by having an honest conversation about the issues and concerns within the relationship. Both parties must be willing to listen and communicate openly.

- Seeking Professional Help: In some cases, seeking the guidance of a therapist or counselor can be instrumental in navigating complex issues and improving communication.

- Setting Boundaries: Establish clear boundaries that respect the needs and expectations of both parties. This can help prevent future conflicts.

- Commitment to Change: Commit to making the necessary changes individually and as a couple. This may involve personal growth, compromise, and forgiveness.

Repairing a relationship is not always easy, but it can be incredibly rewarding if both parties are willing to put in the effort and work together towards a healthier future.

2. Improve

Improving a relationship is a less intensive option than repairing, as it focuses on enhancing the already positive aspects of the relationship. This option is suitable when the foundation of the relationship is strong, but there is room for growth and development. To improve a relationship:

- Acknowledge Strengths: Recognize and celebrate the strengths of the relationship. This positive reinforcement can create a more optimistic atmosphere.

- Quality Time: Spend quality time together, engaging in activities that bring joy and strengthen your bond.

- Continuous Learning: Invest in personal growth and relationship skills to become a better partner.

- Appreciation: Express appreciation and gratitude regularly. Small gestures can have a significant impact on relationship satisfaction.

Improvement is an ongoing process that can lead to a deeper connection and greater satisfaction within the relationship.

3. Leave

Sometimes, despite your best efforts, a relationship may not be salvageable or healthy to maintain. Leaving is a valid choice when the relationship is toxic, abusive, or no longer aligns with your values and well-being. When considering leaving a relationship:

- Safety First: Prioritize your safety, especially in cases of abuse or danger. Seek help from authorities or support networks if necessary.

- Reflect on Boundaries: Revisit your boundaries and values to ensure that your decision aligns with your personal growth and happiness.

- Support System: Lean on friends, family, or therapy for emotional support and guidance during this challenging time.

- Closure: Whenever possible, seek closure by having a respectful and honest conversation with the other party.

Leaving a relationship can be one of the most difficult decisions to make, but it can also be liberating and essential for personal growth and well-being.

In conclusion, making decisions about relationships is a complex and deeply personal process. Evaluating the relationship and exploring options—whether to repair, improve, or leave—requires careful consideration of the specific circumstances and individual needs. Ultimately, the goal is to prioritize your well-being, happiness, and personal growth, while also respecting the feelings and needs of others involved. The journey of decision-making in relationships is a profound and transformative aspect of human existence, shaping the course of our lives and our pursuit of fulfillment and happiness.

CHAPTER 14

Conclusion

14.1 The Importance of Self-Care

14.2 Moving Forward and Learning from Red Flags

Certainly, let's delve into the conclusion regarding the importance of self-care and the significance of learning from red flags. These two topics are deeply interconnected, as self-care plays a pivotal role in recognizing and addressing those red flags that can signal potential issues in our lives. In this conclusion, we'll explore why self-care is essential and how it can empower us to move forward while being vigilant about red flags.

14.1 The Importance of Self-Care

Self-care is a term that has gained significant attention in recent years, and for good reason. It encompasses a wide range of practices and activities that are undertaken with the intention of improving and maintaining our mental, emotional, and physical well-being. Self-care is not merely a luxury; it is a necessity in our fast-paced, often stressful lives.

One of the fundamental aspects of self-care is the act of prioritizing oneself. It involves recognizing that our own needs and well-being are just as important as those of others. This realization is crucial, as neglecting self-care can lead to burnout, diminished mental health, and even physical health issues. In essence, self-care is the foundation upon which our ability to thrive is built.

Self-care takes many forms. It can be as simple as taking a few minutes each day to practice mindfulness or engage in deep breathing exercises. It can also involve more substantial commitments, such as dedicating time to regular exercise, maintaining a balanced diet, or seeking therapy or counseling when needed. The key is to find what works best for you and to make self-care a consistent part of your routine.

Moreover, self-care extends beyond the individual. It has a ripple effect that impacts not only our own lives but also those around us. When we prioritize self-care, we become better equipped to handle the challenges life throws our way. We are more patient, compassionate, and resilient. This not only benefits us but also our relationships, both personal and professional.

In the context of red flags, self-care plays a critical role in our ability to recognize and respond to warning signs. When we are attuned to our own well-being, we are more likely to notice when something doesn't feel right. This heightened awareness can help us identify red flags in various aspects of our lives, such as relationships, work, or our own mental and emotional state.

14.2 Moving Forward and Learning from Red Flags

Red flags are warning signals, indicators that something may be amiss or heading in the wrong direction. They are not to be ignored but rather seen as opportunities for introspection and action. Learning from red flags is a skill that can lead to personal growth, resilience, and ultimately, a more fulfilling life.

One common area where red flags often appear is in relationships. Whether it's a romantic partnership, a friendship, or a professional collaboration, red flags can manifest as behavior or situations that raise concerns. These may include consistent dishonesty, a lack of respect, or a pattern of unfulfilled promises. Recognizing these signs early on can prevent us from investing time and energy in relationships that are ultimately detrimental to our well-being.

In the workplace, red flags can be equally important. They might manifest as signs of burnout, an unhealthy work environment, or a lack of alignment between our values and the organization's culture. Ignoring these signals can lead to increased stress, decreased job satisfaction, and even adverse health effects. Learning from workplace red flags can empower us to make informed decisions about our careers and seek out opportunities that better align with our values and goals.

When it comes to personal well-being, red flags often emerge as symptoms of stress, anxiety, or depression. These can include changes in sleep patterns, loss of interest in activities, or feelings of hopelessness. Acknowledging these signs and seeking support from mental health professionals is a crucial step in managing and overcoming such challenges.

In conclusion, self-care and learning from red flags are two vital components of a healthy and fulfilling life. Self-care provides the foundation for our well-being, enabling us to be more attuned to red flags in various aspects of our lives. Recognizing and responding to red flags empowers us to make informed decisions, protect our well-being, and create a life that aligns with our values and aspirations.

Remember, self-care is not selfish; it is a necessary investment in ourselves that allows us to be our best selves for both our own benefit and the benefit of those around us. Red flags, on the other hand, are not obstacles to be feared but valuable signposts on our life's journey. By embracing self-care and learning from red flags, we can navigate life's challenges with greater resilience and wisdom, ultimately leading to a more fulfilling and purposeful existence.

www.ingramcontent.com/pod-product-compliance
Lightning Source LLC
Chambersburg PA
CBHW070116010626
45794CB00013B/2325